Insprie
Yourself

Vishwamitra Sharma

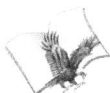

V&S PUBLISHERS

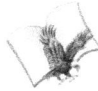

Published by:

V&S PUBLISHERS

F-2/16, Ansari road, Daryaganj, New Delhi-110002
☎ 23240026, 23240027 • *Fax:* 011-23240028
Email: info@vspublishers.com • *Website:* www.vspublishers.com

Regional Office : Hyderabad
5-1-707/1, Brij Bhawan (Beside Central Bank of India Lane)
Bank Street, Koti, Hyderabad - 500 095
☎ 040-24737290
E-mail: vspublishershyd@gmail.com

Branch Office : Mumbai
Jaywant Industrial Estate, 1st Floor–108, Tardeo Road
Opposite Sobo Central Mall, Mumbai – 400 034
☎ 022-23510736
E-mail: vspublishersmum@gmail.com

Follow us on:

Printed at Repro Knowledgecast Limited, Thane

Contents

INDUSTRIALISTS & ENTREPRENEURS

SCIENTISTS

MISCELLANEOUS

Preface

Undoubtedly the cradle of the first major civilisation, five millennia ago India was a fabled land where milk and honey flowed freely. Through the next few millennia, the land produced many noble souls who kept the country's rich spiritual and cultural heritage throbbing. From astronomy, mathematics and medicine to spiritual mastery and renowned universities, the land produced the best in all spheres.

Somewhere down the line, we lost our way, with complacency and inertia taking over, even as the world forged ahead and we were enslaved by different foreign invaders, including the British.

Centuries of serfdom, strife and struggle followed, as we sought to assert our identity and preserve the nation's rich cultural heritage. It was during this period of enslavement that countless inspiring personalities came to the helm, exhorting countrymen to awake from their slumber, throw off the foreign yoke and reclaim India's rightful place among the comity of nations. One man who inspired Indians and foreigners through his oratory was 19th Century legend, Swami Vivekananda, who once said: "First reform yourself before you reform the world."

Once freedom was won, the war was still not over. Centuries of foreign domination had bankrupted the nation and its treasury and the 'Made in India' tag carried negative connotations. A new crop of individuals then came to the fore, ensuring the country did not lag behind in innovation and entrepreneurial spirit. JRD Tata, MS Oberoi, GD Birla, AB Godrej, Jamnalal Bajaj, Jagadish Chandra Bose, CV Raman, Homi Bhabha, Dhirubhai Ambani and others ensured that India's ancient spirit of enterprise was re-ignited. And a guru like Osho Rajneesh showed the path of spiritual freedom not just to Indians but also to foreigners.

Where once we did not manufacture even a safety pin, India is today the cynosure of all eyes with the world's largest pool of trained manpower. In many spheres, the 'Made in India' tag is now flaunted, not hidden – particularly in Information Technology. Where once Indian students aspired to study at Oxford, Cambridge, Stanford and other foreign universities, today the best foreign companies come to India every year for bodyshopping at the IIT campuses, vying for our best brains through stupendous packages!

In this amazing turnaround, hundreds and thousands of Indians have played a key role. Selecting only few names has been an arduous task, with other equally deserving ones having been left out due to space constraints. This is not just a collection of achievements and milestones by select individuals – it is the story of an entire era.

I am grateful to M/s V&S Publishers for accepting this book for publication. Thanks also to Ms A Sunita Purushottaman for helping me in this endeavour. And grateful thanks to the editorial staff without whose untiring efforts this book would not have seen the light of day.

–Vishwamitra Sharma
C-3/58, Lawrence Road
Delhi – 110 035
Tel: 27194317

Industrialists and Entrepreneurs

JRD Tata

Industrialist and Visionary

(1904–1993)

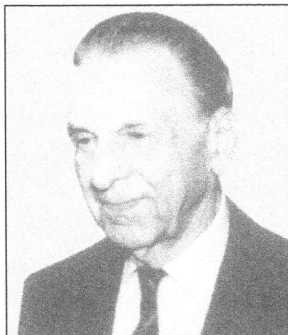

JRD Tata is considered an eminent personality and industrialist of the past Century. He belongs to India's leading family of industrialists who pioneered the country's industrial development. The acumen and foresight that he displayed led to such sustained growth of Tata Industries that one is forced to make a study of the conglomerate. When JRD Tata became the chairman of the Tata Group, it had just 15 companies. Because of his planning the Tata Group grew into 100 companies.

The Tata Group has diversified into a number of areas and is totally engrossed in the service of the people through its hospitals and other service centres.

Jehangir Ratanji Dadabhoy Tata or simply JRD Tata was born on 29 July 1904 in Paris. He was also educated in Paris. In 1938, after the death of Sir Naoroji Saklatvala, one of the nephews of the founders of the company, JRD Tata took over as the chairman of the Tata Group.

JRD Tata was the first Indian to have gained the permission and licence to fly an aeroplane. He first flew from Karachi to Bombay in 1929. There were no special provisions at airports in those days. When he flew from Karachi, the area around the airport was full of ditches. In 1930, he went on a solo flight from Bombay to England on a single-seater aeroplane. And then he founded Tata Airlines in 1932. In 1953, when the race for nationalisation was on, Tata Airlines was nationalised and split into Indian Airlines Corporation, the country's domestic air service, and Air-India, the international carrier.

After JRD took over the reins in 1938, Tata Group took huge strides. He used to trust his people a lot. And some of his most trusted men were S. Mulgaonkar who looked after TELCO, Darbari Seth of Tata Chemicals, Ajit Kerkar who looked after the Taj Group of Hotels, and Russi Modi of TISCO. These were some of the prominent personalities who steered the Tata Group of Industries to staggering heights.

JRD Tata was one of the closest associates of Pt Nehru. However, in spite of this amiable relationship between them, JRD never hesitated to convey his displeasure to Pt Nehru if he found any of the latter's plans inappropriate.

He used to say that he often had to part with people with whom he was closely associated. He knew that whoever came into this world had to depart one day. He was closely associated with the head of the Indian Nuclear Centre, Dr Homi Bhabha. JRD expressed the above thoughts when Dr Homi Bhabha died in an aircrash while returning from Vienna.

The secret of JRD's success was that he did every task with complete dexterity. And this was one of the reasons he was chosen the adviser to a number of committees formed by the government. If he felt that the decisions taken by the government or other committees were inappropriate, he would put forth his view on the subject with such conviction that the other members had no choice but to abide by his wishes.

He not only expanded the Tata empire, but did a lot for the welfare of the people. He set up some of the finest hospitals. In 1992, the government honoured him with the Bharat Ratna.

The ancestors of JRD Tata came to India from Iran when they were being forced to convert to Islam. One of his ancestors Jamshedji Nusserwanji was a man with foresight who set up a steel industry at Jamshedpur and started the industrial revolution. Today Tata Group of Industries is one of the top industrial houses of India.

JRD Tata died on 29 November 1993 in Geneva, Switzerland at the of age of 89.

Ghanshyam Das Birla

Founder of the Birla Group

(1894–1983)

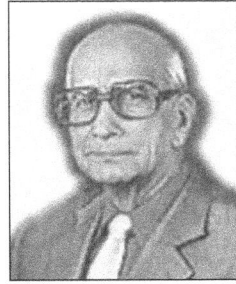

Apart from being an indomitable personality in the industrial field, Ghanshyam Das Birla had many other special qualities. There has been no industrial baron in India who not only found success in his business, but also strode the field of politics with the same poise and confidence. And this was not all. Ghanshyam Das Birla initiated a number of programmes for the betterment of society. He said that earning money was not as difficult as choosing the right way to spend it. He built many temples where people could find solace and peace.

When we look at his entire life in retrospect, we come to the conclusion that he was different from other industrialists. One proof is that he started an industry at a time when the Europeans had a firm hold on Indian industries. And he started some other industries which no one had thought of before.

Ghanshyam Das Birla had an elementary education in arithmetic and Hindi. His father, BD Birla, then initiated him into the world of business in Calcutta. The city was becoming the centre of the jute industry and the British had total control over it. In 1912, his father-in-law, M. Somani, helped him start a brokerage business. Birla was just about 15 or 16. He had come over to Calcutta from Pilani village in Rajasthan. He stayed in the one-room tenement for a long time. He had to sleep, eat, drink, bathe and pray in that room itself.

He established Birla Brothers in 1918. Soon he bought an old cloth mill in Delhi and later diversified into jute. In 1921 he established a cotton mill in Gwalior and in 1923–24 he bought the Keshoram Cotton Mills. By 1939, Birla Brothers made such progress that they were ranked among the top dozen industrialists of those times.

In many areas of business, they ended the dominance of the English and established new industries. The establishment of jute industries is one such example. In connection with the establishment of HINDALCO, he said that he had to undergo a lot of trouble to establish the company and also had to face many problems with the bureaucracy. On the other hand, he was receiving invitations from countries like England and Germany, which wanted him to be a part of their country's development plans. At that time Birla was 60 years old and he felt that he did not want to set industries overseas. He was also of the opinion that aid from the government should not be sought for the establishment of industries.

Birla was actively involved in the freedom struggle and social welfare activities. Gandhiji not only considered Ghanshyam Das Birla his friend, but also a significant adviser. In this way Birla became a link between the British and Gandhiji for talks and advice on matters of India's welfare. Birla also started 400 primary schools in a span of just one year. The driving force behind this endeavour was probably the fact that he himself never had the opportunity to receive proper education. He established the Birla Science Institute in Pilani.

A peek into his life reveals that his way of thinking was different from traditional business people. His approach was modern. But he also listened to the arguments of his critics.

Although he believed in casteism, his life is proof enough that he fully cooperated with the welfare programmes initiated by Gandhiji for the betterment of Harijans. He founded the Harijan Sevak Sangh and remained the president of the institution for many years. In those days, Indians who went abroad had to do penance. Birla opposed this orthodox custom. He, in fact, broke a number of Marwari traditions. On 30 January 1948, Gandhiji was assassinated at Birla House in New Delhi. So Birla dedicated that property to the nation.

G.D. Birla passed away on 11 June 1983, while on a visit to London.

Dhirubhai Ambani

Founder of the Reliance Group

(1932–2002)

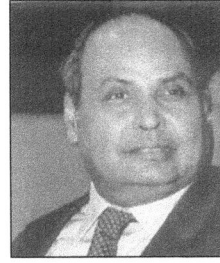

Dhirajlal Hirachand Ambani had expanded his business empire to such dizzy heights in the 20th Century and benefited so many shareholders that other industrialists, wealthy barons and brokers felt threatened. The story of Dhirubhai Ambani is a typical rags-to-riches story. Rising from a room in a chawl to lead the establishment of a big business empire is almost like a wish fulfilled by the genie of Aladdin's lamp.

Dhirubhai Ambani was born on 28 December 1932 in Chorwad, Gujarat. In 1949 at the age of just 17, he went to Aden (now a part of Yemen) and worked for A Besse & Co, the sole distributor of Shell. In 1958 he returned to Bombay (now Mumbai) and started Reliance Commercial Corporation. Armed with only a high school degree, he established the Reliance company, a commodity trading and export house. In 1966 he started a textile mill in Naroda, Ahmedabad.

In 1977 Reliance went public. Then it had 58,000 investors. It rose to over four million equity holders. And this is all because of his intelligence and a special way of working, which had till now never been realised by other industrialists. He has also given a new direction to the Indian economic scenario. He devised a new method of collecting money from the share market on lower interest rates when other companies were taking loans from banks on high interest rates.

In 1991, the Rs 9,000-crore Hazira gas cracker plant was commissioned. Reliance diversified into infrastructure. The following year Reliance became the first Indian company to raise money in global markets with a GDR issue. In 1993 Reliance expanded into plastics and PVC. In 1994 major expansion plans for the Hazira plant were announced. Reliance became the first Indian company to touch net profits of Rs 1,000 crore. In 1996 the company diversified into power and telecom services. The following year the world's largest multi-feed cracker was commissioned in Hazira. Reliance also became the first Asian firm to raise a 100-year debt. It also began cellular services the same year. In 1999 the world's largest grassroot refinery was commissioned at Jamnagar, Gujarat.

In 1986 when he suffered a stroke, his sons Mukesh and Anil were entrusted with additional responsibility of the company.

Some Indian scholars firmly believe in the saying: *Bhagya Phalti Sarvada Na Vidya Na Cha Kausalam.* (Luck helps to prosper rather than sound education or expertise.) But it seems that the baron of Reliance Industries has proved them all wrong. His father was a Gujarati school teacher. Rising from humble beginnings, he scaled new heights and converted his small business into a force to be reckoned with in the international arena. The expansion of the Ambani empire has solely been the result of his intellect and expertise.

In 2001 he received the ET Award for Corporate Excellence for Lifetime Achievement. In 2002 Reliance Petrochemicals merged with Reliance Industries Limited.

Dhirubhai Ambani has been voted as the 'Indian Businessman of the Century' by a worldwide multimedia poll conducted between August and October 1999 by Business Barons.

Dhirubhai Ambani died on 6 July 2002 after suffering a cerebral stroke. Reliance is now an over Rs three lac crore conglomerate.

Mohan Singh Oberoi

The Grand Hotelier

(1898–2002)

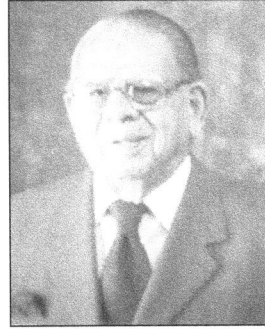

Legendary hotelier Mohan Singh Oberoi officially declared that he was born in 1900 because he did not want to be known as a person of the 19th Century. And when he died in 2002, many said that he was a man of the 21st Century.

What began as a dream in Rawalpindi culminated with the Oberoi chain of hotels comprising 35 hotels in seven countries. But the young teenager dared to dream and what is more significant is that he realised his dream.

MS Oberoi was born on 15 August 1898 in Bhaun. He had to leave his village to pursue further studies. Having failed the examination, he was taking a stroll on the Mall in Shimla when he came across the imposing Hotel Cecil. He asked for a job in the hotel and he was given the job of a clerk with a salary of Rs 50 per month. That was his break into the hospitality business.

Dame Luck smiled on him and a series of promotions and a switch of job later, he was working as the manager of Hotel Clarkes. It was then that Ernest Clarke, the owner of Hotel Clarkes, decided to move over to England. So in 1934, he mortgaged his wife's jewellery and with some financial help from an elderly uncle, he acquired the Clarkes Hotel from Mr Clarke for Rs 20,000.

In 1938, he acquired the 500-room Grand Hotel on a lease of Rs 8,000 per month. The city was then reeling from an outbreak of cholera. During the Second World War, the Allied troops sought refuge in the hotel. The British were pleased with his hospitality and bestowed upon him the title Rai Bahadur. Soon he made a string of acquisitions – even Hotel Flashmans, the hotel that inspired him to dream big. His first international venture was Soaltee Oberoi in Nepal in 1969.

Oberoi Group of Hotels now has a chain of five-star hotels in Melbourne, Bali, Colombo, Mauritius, Cairo, Budapest, among others. The Oberoi Group was the first to employ women in hotels.

Oberoi was elected to the Rajya Sabha twice – in 1962 and 1972, and once to the Lok Sabha in 1968. He was honoured with the Padma Bhushan in 2001. *Newsweek* named him one of its 'Elite Winners of 1978' for his valuable contribution to the world of business.

Once when he was asked what motivated him, he said, "The idea was never merely to make money. The compulsion was to think big, always to offer the best." When Oberoi turned 100, the Oberoi Group of Hotels had a range of heritage properties across the world including Melbourne's Windsor Hotel and Oberoi Maidens in India, which is a heritage building.

He once said, "I have been able to accept the challenge and make good – there is comfort in knowing that whatever little I have achieved has also helped to raise the prestige of my country." He made the best out of the opportunities and that is the secret of his success.

Ramnath Goenka

The Fearless Newspaper Baron

(1904–1991)

Ramnath Goenka was the only newspaper baron who opposed Indira Gandhi during the Emergency period. During the Emergency, not only was Goenka's Delhi office raided, all efforts were made to put an end to his empire. But Goenka thwarted these efforts with valour. The reigns of the government were in the hands of Indira Gandhi and she wielded a lot of power, but that did not deter him from opposing Indira's government. This was the first time in the history of independent India that an individual had stood up to the government.

He was born on 3 April 1904 in Darbhanga in Bihar.

Most newspapers and media personalities adopted the middle path rather than invite the wrath of the government. But Goenka refused to bow down before the whims and fancies of the government. And he emerged a winner. When India went to the polls, Indira Gandhi was badly defeated and the Janata Party came to power.

The Janata Party lauded Goenka's steadfastness. But Goenka never tried to take undue advantage of this proximity to the ruling party.

Along with the English edition of the *Indian Express*, he also brought out newspapers in Hindi and regional languages like *Jansatta* and *Loksatta*. He also published the film journal *Screen*. S. Mulgaonkar, S. Gurumurthy and Arun Shourie were some of the prominent journalists who worked for him.

Ramnath Goenka was born in a Marwari family in Darbhanga (Bihar) and was religious-minded. He went on pilgrimage to Tirupati frequently. Goenka started *Indian Express* in 1932, but he became more well known during the Emergency.

Ramnath Goenka died on 5 October 1991 in Mumbai.

N.R. Narayana Murthy

Founder of Infosys

(Born 1946)

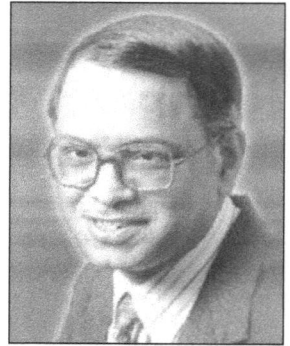

Narayana Murthy is the founder of one of the world's most successful software giants. What is remarkable is not that the company and its business is extensive, but the fact that the company functions with a lot of discernment. As a result, when a majority of the software companies are trying to make a mark in the international arena, Murthy's company, Infosys, is conducting most of its business abroad.

Narayana Murthy started the company in 1981 along with six close associates. For some time the company's annual turnover remained Rs 50 crores, but what is remarkable is that America chose Murthy's company as the first Indian company for its trade relations. Apart from the home front, even Nasdaq, which is considered the Mecca of high-level technical companies, has rated Infosys as a top-level software company. The secret of the success of Infosys and Narayana Murthy is that they plunged into the business of computers and information technology when the time was ripe.

Narayana Murthy studied electrical engineering from Mysore University. Then he joined IIT, Kanpur for a degree in computer science. Murthy comes from a humble background. His father was a school teacher in the Kolar district of Karnataka.

It was because of his acumen that he reached such a position where his profits soared from Rs 117 million to Rs 293.52 million. The income generated outside the country increased from Rs 500 million to Rs 869 million. The company is progressing by leaps and bounds and its net worth runs into hundreds of billions.

Sabeer Bhatia

The Young Achiever

(Born 1966)

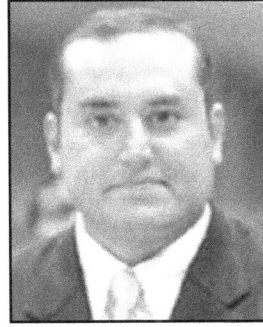

At the age of 45, the achievement of Sabeer Bhatia is remarkable. He has not only made a name for himself, but has also acquired a lot of wealth. Sabeer Bhatia's 'Hotmail' has changed the lives of people the world over. What is astounding is the fact that when he got started with 'Hotmail', he just had three clients. Today it caters to more than 220 million people worldwide.

The momentous occasion in Sabeer Bhatia's life came when Microsoft decided to buy 'Hotmail' for $400 million. This catapulted Sabeer Bhatia to fame and fortune overnight.

Bhatia was born in Chandigarh. In 1984, he joined the California Institute of Technology in the US for higher studies. Then he went to Stanford to do his Masters in electronic engineering. He tried his hand at various jobs, but the critical point in his life came in 1996 when he started 'Hotmail' along with Jack Smith of Apple Computers. After he sold 'Hotmail', Sabeer started a new company called Arzoo.com. This was shut down in June 2001 due to the downturn in business.

Men like Sabeer Bhatia have not only made a mark for themselves, but also made India proud.

Shiv Nadar

IT Entrepreneur

(Born 1945)

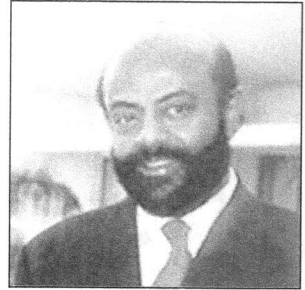

Among the world's renowned people connected with the world of information technology, Shiv Nadar is considered one of the greatest entrepreneurs in the field of computers. In 1975, when the whole of India had just 250 computers, he established the company HCL. Now the company has 19 branches outside India. There are a total of 30 branches of HCL and the annual turnover of the company is over 4700 million dollars. This is proof enough that Shiv Nadar worked with a lot of prudence.

In 1997, *Time* magazine praised him for his perception and rationality.

What puts Shiv Nadar apart from other industrialists is that he had the right perception about the market and could rightly guess the pulse of the international market. In his book, *Giant Killer*, Geoffrey James puts Shiv Nadar's company HCL at par with Microsoft, Hewlitt-Packard and Compaq. This tells us that his company is no less than these giant blue chip companies.

Nadar studied electronic engineering from Coimbatore and started as a system analyst. He also worked with the Delhi Cloth Mills as chief administrator. Then he established HCL. Shiv Nadar believes in the proverb 'Strike when the iron is hot'.

Harprasad Nanda

Pioneering Industrialist

(1917–1999)

Harprasad Nanda was one of the pioneers to establish industries after the independence of India. Before the partition of the country, he had established the Escorts Group of Industries at Lahore in 1944, but after Partition, he lost all his wealth and so re-established the industries in Delhi.

Harprasad Nanda was born on 9 January 1917 in Jammu. When he wanted to revive the Escorts Group in India, he was short of finances, but with his dedication, intelligence and truthfulness, he progressed. Initially, he set up a factory in Faridabad for the manufacture of agricultural implements and tractors. Then he began the manufacture of Rajdoot motorcycles. Now his company Escorts is a well known and popular brand name.

Harprasad Nanda will also be remembered for the whole-hearted determination with which he opposed the attempt of London-based NRI businessman Swraj Paul to buy off the shares of Escorts and take over the company in 1983.

Escorts Group of Companies is being looked after by his sons Rajan and Anil. Nanda's son Rajan is married to the daughter of the famous film producer and actor, the late Raj Kapoor.

Harprasad Nanda's name has been etched in the pages of history as one of the pioneering industrialists of independent India.

Laxman Rao Kirloskar

Powering the Nation

(1869–1956)

The word 'Kirloskar' brings to mind the whirring sound produced by power generators. Laxman Rao Kirloskar is one of the few industrialists who identified the fact that apart from developing the state of agriculture, it was necessary to simultaneously develop industrial strength for the welfare of the country. He felt that for the development of villages it was imperative that we invent the right tools and implements.

So initially he developed the iron plough to replace the wooden one. The plough was the primary tool used by a farmer, and a wooden one had to be replaced every year. But an iron one could last a lifetime. However, procuring the iron was a problem. So he bought old iron cannons from the King of Kolhapur.

The Kirloskar company now manufactures a number of agricultural and engineering equipment and engines. These play an important role in industries. In this way Kirloskar had a far-reaching impact on these industries. He paid attention to the fact that the machines manufactured by him were the best in quality. As a result, not only in India, he was highly respected in the world too. And this respect he earned in 1926 itself.

In 1926, he held an exhibition of his products. Many people including foreigners had seen the products for the first time. And one of them asked whether the goods were of foreign origin.

Even after so many years the capacity and quality of Kirloskar engines and other equipments have not lessened. The Kirloskar group has recently started an automobile plant for the manufacture of cars.

Laxman Rao Kirloskar's name has been etched forever among the prominent industrialists of the 20th Century.

Karsanbhai Patel

The 'Nirma' Man

(Born 1943)

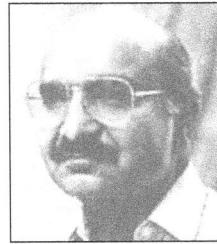

There are some consumer products that have become an integral part of our life. One such product is Nirma detergent powder. There are a number of detergent powders in the market including those marketed by multinationals. But the total sales of all the other detergent powders combined is less than half the sales of Nirma. This makes it clear that the manufacturer of Nirma, Karsanbhai Patel, has displayed immense shrewdness. His life proves that if a person works hard, it is not difficult to put an idea into practice and become a success.

In 1966, Karsanbhai was working at a factory in Ahmedabad as a chemist and drawing a salary of Rs 150 per month. He found it hard to make both ends meet. So in his spare time he made detergent powder at home and went from door to door on his cycle selling his product. Soon he thought of expanding his business. So he began to sell the powder in packets. He had started a factory in the backyard of his home. Soon he began to supply the detergent to various shops in Ahmedabad. Nirma gradually became popular not only in small towns, but also in big cities. Karsanbhai's product soon made its presence felt in the Indian market. Thus Karsanbhai was able to expand his business all over the country in a short span of time.

The secret of Karsanbhai's success is that he made quality products available for the average customer at competitive prices. Consumers realised that instead of using a bar of detergent to scrub and clean dirty clothes, it was better to keep them soaked in a good and cheaper detergent. This compelled the multinational Hindustan Lever to rethink its products, strategies and policies. Today Nirma products are household names and the company's networth is around Rs.3000 crore.

Keshub Mahindra

Progressive Industrialist

(Born 1923)

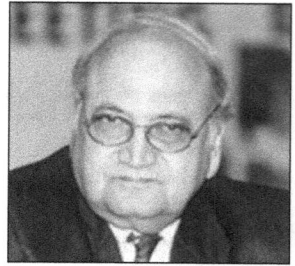

Keshub Mahindra is the chairman of Mahindra & Mahindra Group of Companies. He is one of those 15 top industrialists whose age is above 75 years and one of those 10 industrialists who command a great deal of respect in the industrial world.

Mahindra & Mahindra manufactures jeeps and other vehicles which have found a place in the consumer market because of their quality and sturdiness. The vehicles are all-terrain vehicles.

Keshub Mahindra was born in Shimla. He is one of those accomplished industrialists who has not only seen the industrial progress of five decades of his company, but was also the chairman of various companies like Union Carbide, Indian Aluminium, Remington Red and Otis Elevators.

Mahindra & Mahindra Group, which was established in 1947, made quick progress. Apart from tractors, the company also manufactures other vehicles. He believed that for being successful, it was necessary that one should be organised and work in coordination. It was because of his wisdom and expertise that he is one of the leading industrialists of India.

Azim H. Premji

The Wipro Legend

(Born 1945)

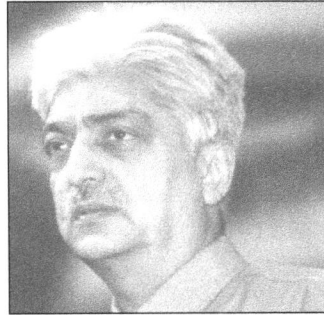

India occupies a significant position in the world of Information Technology. And the most prominent company in the field of IT is Azim H. Premji's Bangalore-based company, Wipro Corporation.

Azim Hasham Premji was born in Bombay in 1945. His father owned a cooking fat manufacturing company by the name Western India Vegetable Products Ltd (Wipro). Azim Premji graduated in engineering from Stanford University. And when he returned to India in 1966, he had to take over the family business because of his father's death. Premji was a man with a vision. Instead of venturing into industrial production, he focused on consumer preferences and needs. He used attractive packaging to woo consumers and further the Wipro brand name. He also did away with middlemen and sold his products directly to the consumer, thereby increasing his profits. Contrary to other family-run businesses, he did not appoint members of his own family, but recruited management and engineering graduates. He diversified his business into bath soaps, hydraulic fluid, electrical appliances, baby products and finance

In 1979, the American computer giant Internationl Business Machines (IBM) was denied permission to continue its operations in the country. This was when Premji ventured into computers. Soon his company became one of the world's biggest computer manufacturing companies. Then he ventured into software development, which alone accounts for a considerable portion of his company's annual sales.

With an estimated personal wealth of $35 billion, Azim Premji is one of the world's richest men.

Sir Shri Ram

Famous Industrialist

(1883–1963)

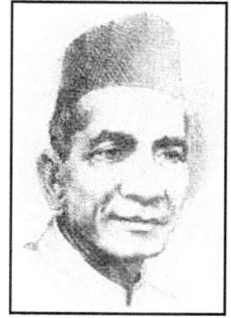

Sir Shri Ram started his career as an assistant secretary in the Delhi Cloth & General Mills, on a salary of rupees one hundred per month. By the time he died, he was one of the noted industrialists of the country. He got the job in Delhi Cloth Mills only because his father Madan Mohan was also working there.

Delhi Cloth Mills was at that time owned by the Gurwala family. Gurwala was a money-lender to the Nawab of Avadh and the Mughals in 1857. The family was ruined during the Bank Crises of 1913. At that time, even a prominent bank like People's Bank closed down. The Delhi Cloth Mills also passed through a great crisis in 1917. However, it managed to survive when it got orders to manufacture tents for the British Army during the First World War.

It is to the credit of Sir Shri Ram that he brought this Cloth Mill into the forefront of north Indian mills. Sir Shri Ram was an able administrator. He had great knowledge of raw materials and cotton which was required for his mill. His idol was Tata. He engaged retired civil servants like Dr Dharamveer in the management of the mill. Dr Dharamveer had occupied prominent government posts when in service.

In 1930, he established a sugar mill in Daurala, UP. Today many diversified concerns of Delhi Cloth Mills are spread over various places in India, prominent among them being Bengal Potteries, Jai Engineering Works, Usha Sewing Machines, Shri Ram Fertilisers, etc. It was diligent, untiring hard work, iron will-power and great ambition that enabled a man, who himself once earned Rs100 a month, to employ thousands of people.

Ardeshir Burjorji Godrej

Founder of the Godrej Empire

(1868–1936)

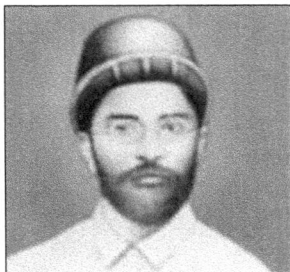

Among the builders of modern Indian industry, Ardeshir Burjorji Godrej, the founder of the Godrej Group, was a true innovator, a pioneer and a visionary.

Innovation was born out of his innate desire to be a *swadeshi* manufacturer. But *swadeshi* did not merely mean boycott of British goods. It meant utilising one's resources and genius to create something that was truly Indian. Driven by patriotic passion, Godrej began to work on a commodity that was to make Godrej a household name: the lock. Ardeshir Burjorji Godrej was born in Broach on 26 March 1868. He was educated in Bombay, and was a practising lawyer. Once he went to Zanzibar to plead a case for his client. He argued well but at a particular point, in order to win the case for his client, he had to twist the facts, which he found immoral and unethical. He not only lost the case but also bade farewell to the legal profession.

During the first decade of the 20th Century, the nationalist leaders gave a call for *swadeshi* and boycott. Ardeshir pleaded with the Indian leaders that the political battle even if won, would not amount to much so long as we were in the bondage of industrial slavery. India had to become economically self-reliant, otherwise freedom would remain a distant dream. He argued that in order to achieve this, instead of depending on goods manufactured abroad, we had to utilise our own manpower, establish our own industry and use our own raw materials.

He therefore decided to start manufacturing surgical instruments in India. The problem, however, was the capital. He required a few thousand rupees and he didn't have the money. Then, he approached Merwanji Cama, a multimillionaire and asked for a loan. Mr Cama readily obliged and gave him a few thousand rupees. Ardeshir manufactured the surgical instruments and they were up to the mark. The snag, however, was that chemists would not sell surgical instruments made in India and the venture flopped.

A lesser person would have given up the fight but Ardeshir was made of different stuff. He found out that making locks and safes was an ancient art going back 4,000 years and Indian workmen were already preparing locks of different kinds. He studied the technology thoroughly and decided to manufacture locks the likes of which India had never seen before and which would vie with locks imported from foreign countries. Since then, the Godrej family has never looked back. They went from strength to strength selling different varieties of locks and later manufacturing safes and bank lockers.

Ardeshir adopted the latest technology in his factory but in his organisation there was not a single foreigner. When Jawaharlal Nehru visited the factory, he immediately noticed this and wondered how the House of Godrej would carry on without a foreign expert. Ardeshir assured him that he had full faith in the competence of his artisans and they had delivered the goods. Since then, the Godrej family has come a long way, diversified into personal-care products, food processing machine tools, office systems, etc. but the basic principles of honesty, integrity and service have always remained unchanged.

When Ardeshir Godrej went to Merwanji Cama to repay the loan, the latter waived it away. The only stipulation was that he should take his nephew Boyce into the Godrej concern and add his name to the firm. Ardeshir readily agreed. The nephew soon lost interest and dropped out but the name "Boyce" continued.

Having succeeded at making the first rudimentary security system, Godrej opened shop, setting up the Godrej & Boyce Mfg Co in 1897. At a time when the 'Made in England' tag was enough to sell goods, Godrej was able to break the customer's mental barrier.

A Century later, his spirit of innovation still drives his group.

Scientists

Jagadish Chandra Bose

Discoverer of Life in Plants

(1858–1937)

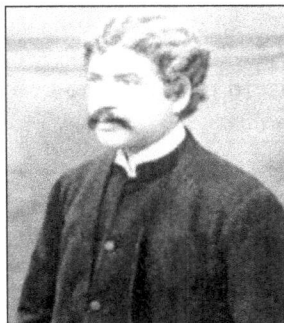

The contribution of Jagadish Chandra Bose cannot be bound by time or Century. He has several firsts to his credit, but he was so engrossed in his work that he never pursued fame.

Dr Jagadish Chandra Bose was a scientist of rare intellect. The extent of work carried out by Bose was significant because no other scientist had done any work in this field. And he will be remembered for another important deed. He always made an attempt to get Indian officials the same respect and salary as their British counterparts. He struggled for three years and was finally successful in getting the same salary as an English professor.

Jagadish Chandra Bose was born in Memansingh district (now in Bangladesh) of West Bengal on 30 November 1858. His father was a collector. At the age of 13, he went to Calcutta (now Kolkata) for higher education and, in 1880, he received admission at Christ College in Cambridge. At Cambridge, he worked with a professor of physics, Roley. It was here that he befriended the famous biologist Dr Vines and became interested in biology.

In 1885, he returned to Calcutta and was appointed professor of physical science at Presidency College.

After dedicating himself to teaching, his interest in conducting research was sparked. In 1915, he left the university to found the Bose Research Institute, Calcutta. He first conducted research on electricity and with the help of wires created waves that made a telephone, which was kept at a distance of 75 feet, ring. His experiment on the quasi-optical properties of very short radio waves led him to make improvements on the cohere, an early form of radio detector, which contributed to the development of solid-state physics. However, in spite of the fact that Bose studied electric waves first, it was Marconi who got the credit.

Dr Bose then switched over to botany and began to study plants very minutely. For his research, he invented a device called the cryocograph. This device measured the development of a plant. He constructed automatic recorders that could register even the slightest movements. He also developed other devices to measure the effect of sleep, air, food and poison. With the help of his research, he concluded that plants also slept, felt joy and pain like other living beings.

Because of his exemplary works, Dr Bose was made a member of the Royal Society of London. He went to England and America a number of times and demonstrated his research with the help of his devices. In 1915, he pooled in all his resources and established the Bose Research Institute. He was able to interest the world's scientists in his work and his fame grew. Rabindranath Tagore remained one of his steadfast friends.

His published works include *Response in the Living and Non-living* and *The Nervous Mechanism of Plants*.

M.S. Swaminathan

Father of the Green Revolution

(Born 1925)

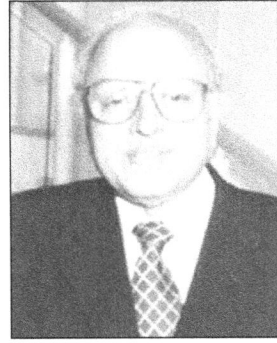

India is a land of villages and a majority of the people are involved in agriculture. However, the land is prone to droughts and famines. During the reign of the British, the people led a very miserable life. Famines were frequent and there was no respite from them. The main reason for the sad plight of the people was that they were using age-old methods of farming. Nobody paid attention to the development of better seeds.

It was Monkombu Sambisivan Swaminathan who first realised that developing better varieties of seeds was the only solution to make India self-reliant in crops. He accepted a variety of the Mexican wheat to solve the Indian crop crisis. This helped increase India's crop production. Therefore, Swaminathan is often referred to as the harbinger of India's Green Revolution. Since then India has become so self-reliant that there has been a steady increase in crop production and the country also exports crops.

Dr Swaminathan was born on 7 August 1925 at Kumbhkonam town in Tamil Nadu in the family of a nationalist doctor, Samishivan Swaminathan. Dr Swaminathan dedicated himself completely to agriculture and agriculture-based projects. For five years he worked with an international rice institute and returned to India in 1988. Then he was appointed the director of Pusa Institute, the director of Indian Agricultural Research Centre, and the Secretary of the Agricultural Ministry.

Along with the Royal Society of London, 14 other prominent international science centres granted him fellowship. Many universities also honoured him with doctorates. In 1967, he was honoured with the Padma Shri and in 1972 with the Padma Bhushan. The country gave accolades to a person who never tried

33

to steal the limelight. In 1971, he also received the Magsaysay Award for Community Leadership. He received the Albert Einstein Award in 1986, the first World Food Prize in 1987, the Tyler Prize of the United States in 1991, Japan's Honda Prize for Eco-technology in 1994, France's *Ordre du Merite Agricole* (Order of Merit in Agriculture) in 1997, the Henry Shaw Medal of the Missouri Botanical Garden (USA) in 1998, the Volvo International Environment Award and the UNESCO Gandhi Gold Award in 1999. In 1999, *Time* magazine voted him one of the 20 most influential Asians of the 20th Century.

Apart from being a well-known agricultural scientist, Dr Swaminathan was also an efficient administrator. He played a significant role in the handling of various plans and projects. Because of his undaunted efforts, India's food problems were resolved and his fame spread. Nobel laureate and famous agricultural scientist Dr Norman E Borlaug has also praised Dr Swaminathan's efforts.

In the early 1990s he established the MS Swaminathan Research Foundation in Madras (now Chennai) with the funds he received from various awards and prizes. The research centre has done pioneering work towards job-led economic growth strategy in Indian villages. It is based on a pro-nature and pro-women orientation to technology development and dissemination of information. The contribution of Swaminathan and the Centre has received international recognition. Swaminathan holds the UNESCO Chair in Eco-technology with Responsibility for South Asia.

If we consider the efforts of Dr Swaminathan in entirety, we will realise that he has made an immense contribution for the development of the rural sector. He was able to inspire the common Indian farmer to accept new farming methods. The country has witnessed a dramatic progress in plant conservation and development, which has resulted in a great revolution in crop production.

Sir C.V. Raman

Prominent Indian Scientist

(1888–1970)

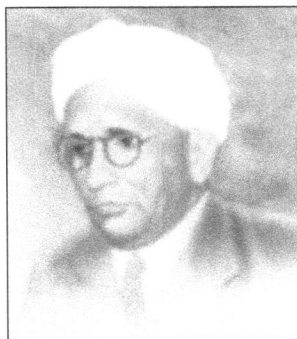

Chandrasekhara Venkata Raman is considered one of those prominent personalities of the 20th Century who was not disturbed by the trials and tribulations in life and remained steadfast, thus becoming successful in achieving his aim. He was the first Indian scientist to win the Nobel Prize for Physics in 1930 for the discovery that when light traverses a transparent medium, some of the light that is deflected changes its wavelength. This phenomenon is now called the Raman Effect.

C.V. Raman was born on 7 November 1880 at Thiruvanaikkaval near Tiruchirappalli, Tamil Nadu into an orthodox South Indian family. He was a brilliant student. At the age of 11 he completed his matriculation. After graduating from Presidency College, Madras (now Chennai) at the age of 15, he wanted to go to England. But he was disqualified on medical grounds. So after acquiring a master's degree in Physics from the college in 1907, Raman joined as an assistant accountant general in the finance department of the Indian Government.

He was posted to Calcutta. It was here that he discovered the Indian Association for the Cultivation of Science, where he began doing his research work, outside office hours. In 1917, Sir Ashutosh Mukherjee appointed him the Palit Professor of Physics at the newly-endowed chair in the Calcutta University.

The turning point of his life came when he had the opportunity to go to Europe in 1921 as a representative of Calcutta University at a science meet. He wondered why the water of the Mediterranean Sea had such a dark shade of blue. Light became the subject of Raman's study. Studying the scattering of light in various substances, in 1928 he discovered that when a beam of light of one frequency illuminates a transparent object

– solid, liquid or gaseous – a small portion of the light emerges at right angles to the original direction, and some of this light is of different frequencies than that of the incident light. These so-called Raman-frequencies are equal to the infrared frequencies for the scattering material and caused by the exchange of energy between the light and the material. His discovery was named the "Raman Effect". He used a mercury arc and a spectrograph for his study.

In 1929, Raman received knighthood. In 1930 he became the first Indian to win the Nobel Prize for Physics. He described his experience thus, "When the Nobel award was announced, I saw it as a personal triumph, an achievement, a recognition for a very remarkable discovery, for reaching the goal I had pursued for seven years. But when I sat in that crowded hall and I saw the sea of western faces surrounding me, and I, the only Indian, in my turban and closed coat, it dawned on me that I was really representing my country and my people. I felt truly humble when I received the prize from King Gustav; it was a moment of great emotion, but I could restrain myself. Then I turned round and saw the British Union Jack under which I had been sitting and it was then that I realised that my poor country, India, did not have even a flag of her own – and it was this that triggered off my complete breakdown."

In 1933, he joined the Indian Institute of Science, Bangalore and served as its director until 1937. Next, he was the head of the department of physics until 1947. Then he retired from the Indian Institute and founded the Raman Research Institute in Bangalore. The land was a gift from the then king of Mysore. He founded the *Indian Journal of Physics* and the Indian Academy of Sciences. He was closely associated with many Indian research institutions of his time.

Raman also did some outstanding research on musical instruments like the violin and the veena. His research on the veena was documented in the work, *On the Mechanical Theory of Vibrations of Musical Instruments of the Violin Family.*

He was honoured with the Bharat Ratna in 1954. In 1957 he won the International Lenin Prize. He died on 21 November 1970 in Bangalore.

Dr Homi Jehangir Bhabha

Father of India's Nuclear Programme

(1909–1966)

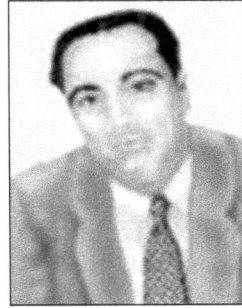

Dr Homi Bhabha was not only India's eminent physicist, he was also the principal architect of India's nuclear programme. Dr Bhabha realised the importance of developing alternate energy sources for India because natural sources were limited. But Pt Nehru felt that in a poor country like India, the priorities of the government were very different from developing nuclear power. It took a lot of convincing by JRD Tata and Homi Bhabha for Pt Nehru to agree to it.

Dr Homi Jehangir Bhabha was born in a rich, aristocratic Parsi family on 30 October 1909 in Bombay. After his formal education in India, he joined the University of Cambridge to study mechanical engineering. After obtaining his degree in 1930, he joined Cavendish Laboratories in Cambridge to carry out research. In 1935, he obtained his doctorate.

He had come to India on a holiday, when the Second World War broke out in Europe. As all of Europe was in turmoil, he decided to stay back in India. It was during his stay in India that he met Nobel laureate Sir C.V. Raman, who was then the director of the Indian Institute of Science, Bangalore. He asked Dr Bhabha to join the institute. So in 1940, Dr Bhabha joined the Indian Institute of Science as a reader in Physics.

Being from an aristocratic family, Dr Bhabha had a western upbringing. But he envisaged a bright future for India. He realised the importance of developing nuclear energy for the industrial growth of India. So in 1945, Bhabha founded the Tata Institute of Fundamental Research (TIFR). The funds were arranged by JRD Tata. In 1948, the Atomic Energy Commission was instituted by the Government of India and Dr Bhabha was appointed its Chairman. He later founded the Atomic Energy Establishment in Trombay.

His contribution towards India's nuclear programme earned him world renown. In 1955, he was appointed the president of the United Nations Conference for Peaceful Uses of Atomic Energy. Between 1960 and 1963, he served as the president of the International Union of Pure and Applied Physics.

However, the eminent physicist died in an air crash over Mont Blanc in the Swiss Alps on 24 January 1966. The Atomic Energy Establishment in Trombay was renamed the Bhabha Atomic Research Centre (BARC) in memory of its founder.

Dr Vikram Sarabhai

Scientist, Industrialist, Educationist

(1919–1971)

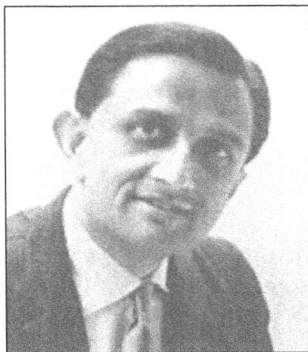

Dr Vikram Sarabhai is called the father of Indian space research. He not only developed Indian rocketry, he developed scientific research centres to carry out research in the field and remained attached to these organisations till the end. From the development of uranium for nuclear energy to the development of rockets and missiles to the installation of nuclear power stations, he was involved in all the projects. Dr Vikram Sarabhai strongly advocated that India should not sign the Non- Proliferation Treaty till the country did not develop nuclear weapons.

Vikram Sarabhai believed that development of science was of utmost importance for the progress of the country. He was aware of all the hurdles that would hinder the growth of the country. For example, he wanted scientists and engineers to come forward and join hands to find a solution for the shortage of water and the problem of droughts in the country.

The contribution made by Dr Sarabhai towards space and nuclear research in the 20th Century is stupendous. He established the Indian Space Research Organisation (ISRO) at Thumba, a remote fishing village near Trivandrum in Kerala and became its first chairman. The centre has developed a number of satellites that have helped India take giant strides in the field of mass communications and weather forecasting.

Vikram Ambalal Sarabhai was born on 12 August 1919, in Ahmedabad into a well-to-do industrialist family. When he was only two years old, Rabindranath Tagore predicted that the child would one day earn a lot of fame and recognition.

Mathematics and science were his favourite subjects. He was also deeply inclined towards physics. In 1936, he completed his Intermediate from Gujarat College, Ahmedabad. In 1936, he joined Cambridge University and in 1939, at the age of 20, he passed the Tripos examination in physics. When the Second World War broke out, he returned to India. Here he had the opportunity of meeting Sir C.V. Raman and undertook research in cosmic rays under his guidance. Once the War was over, he returned to Cambridge to pursue his doctorate and wrote the thesis on *Cosmic Ray Investigations in Tropical Latitudes*. When he came back to India, he founded the Physical Research Laboratory in Ahmedabad.

He also established the Ahmedabad Textile Industries' Research Association (ATIRA) in 1947, which tried to solve technical problems faced by the textile industry. He looked after the centre till 1956. He established Sarabhai Chemicals, the first pharmaceutical company in the country to make basic drugs. It was because of his efforts that the Indian Institute of Management was instituted in 1962. The same year he established the Indian National Committee for Space Research, which was later renamed the Indian Space Research Organisation (ISRO). He also set up the Thumba Equatorial Rocket Launching Station.

Besides being involved in the research of solar radiation in the Physical Research Laboratory at Ahmedabad, he also worked on the development of nuclear energy, software technology, space research, physical sciences and astronomy. He took over as the chairman of the Atomic Energy Commission in 1966, after the death of Dr Homi Bhabha. The development of India's first artificial satellite was done at the Physical Research Laboratory. He encouraged the development of indigenous nuclear technology for defence purposes.

In 1966 he was honoured with the Padma Shri. He died prematurely in his sleep, while visiting Thumba on 30 December 1971. In 1972 he was posthumously awarded the Padma Vibhushan.

Dr M. Visvesvaraya

Engineer, Administrator and Educationist

(1861–1962)

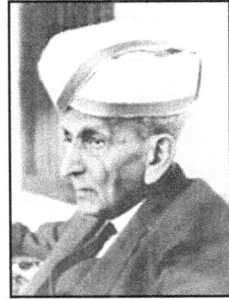

D r Mokshagundam Visvesvaraya always strove for a better tomorrow. In this, he found a friend in Krishnaraj Vadiyar, the King of Mysore. Krishnaraj Vadiyar tried to improve the lot of his subjects with the help of Dr Visvesvaraya. Today, Mysore is a part of Karnataka. In the beginning of the 20th Century, when the rulers of other princely states were indifferent to the plight of their subjects, the King of Mysore took steps to educate his subjects and put the state on the path to industrial progress. He chalked out a number of welfare programmes and entrusted the task of turning his ideas into reality to Dr Visvesvaraya. The duo transformed Mysore into a centre of industrial, agricultural and other strongholds.

Dr Visvesvaraya worked on several irrigation projects in the city. As an engineer, Dr Visvesvaraya also handled many water drainage and irrigation projects in other parts of the country. It is because of his successful projects that Dr Visvesvaraya achieved a place of honour among prominent personalities and was honoured with the Bharat Ratna. His work provided the necessary infrastructure for the industrial growth of India.

Dr Visvesvaraya was born on 15 September 1860 at a village in Chikvalpur district of Mysore. His father Shrinivas Shastri did not have the resources to educate his children, but Dr Visvesvaraya showed signs of ingenuity right from childhood. He gave tuitions to young children to provide for his own education. He obtained a scholarship in college and completed his BSC from Bangalore University with flying colours. Then he joined the Science College at Poona. One advantage of joining the college was that the candidate who stood first in the college was directly appointed as Assistant Engineer in the Public Works Department (PWD).

So Visvesvaraya joined the PWD when he was 23. His fruitful life began from here.

He had the distinction of turning many impossible ideas into reality, because of which he was praised even by British officers. After Bombay, he had the opportunity of working in Nasik. Then he was sent to Khandesh. A perennial river at Dhuliya in Khandesh caused much woe to the people. He not only harnessed the river waters to prevent floods, but also made arrangements to provide safe drinking water for the people of Khandesh. Next, he was entrusted with the task of providing water to Poona and later to the northern part of Sakkhar in Sindh. The project was difficult to accomplish, but under his supervision, manufacturing of tanks and drains was completed on time. The project was to carry waters of the Indus River to a tank built over a mountain and then to the town. When the Governor of Bombay (Sindh was then a part of Bombay) inaugurated the project, he showered Visvesvaraya with praise. Such successful projects made him a well-known figure

So he was promoted to the post of superintending engineer. He then worked on projects in Bangalore, Poona, Mysore, Karachi, Baroda, Gwalior, Indore, Kolhapur, Sangli, Surat, Nasik, Nagpur, Dharwad, Bijapur and other cities and solved the problem of water shortage in these areas.

The King of Mysore, Vadiyar IV, was highly impressed by his works and called him over to Mysore. At first, he appointed Visvesvaraya the chief engineer of his state and later, the *diwan*. He built the Krishnarajsagar dam on the river Cauvery, which provided water for irrigation and for hydro-electricity. This was the first hydro-electrical project in India.

In September 1961, when he had completed 101 years, he was asked the secret of his long life and he exclaimed that the secret was his work being done on time. He also wrote many books that shed light on his projects. One of his books, *Reconstructing India*, is a trendsetting book for architects and builders.

Dr Visvesvaraya died on 14 April 1962 in Bangalore at the age of 101.

Dr Raja Ramanna

Father of the Indian Atomic Bomb

(1925–2004)

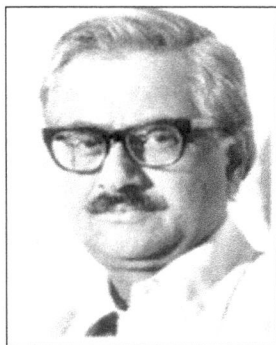

Dr Raja Ramanna is one of the prominent scientists who helped India in making the atom bomb. In the modern age, the potential of the atom bomb cannot be underestimated. Till a few decades, the country had to look up to other nations for all essential supplies. It was in 1944 that Dr Homi Jehangir Bhabha said, "In a few years from now, when we will become successful in producing nuclear energy on a vast scale, we will not be required to look up to others. In fact, we'll prepare our own experts." It was as a result of Dr Bhabha's foresight that we had an expert in nuclear physics like Dr Raja Ramanna. The Tarapur nuclear energy centre was developed because of his efforts.

Ramanna's formal education was completed in Mysore. Then he went to Bangalore and Madras for further studies. After completing his Intermediate from St Joseph's College in Bangalore, Ramanna joined Christian College in Madras for his BSc (Hons.) in Physics. After MSc, he went to King's College, London for his PhD in Molecular (Nuclear) Physics. After completing his PhD in 1948, he started his research for DSc. In 1949, he joined the Tata Institute of Fundamental Research in Bombay as a professor. In 1953, he joined Bhabha Atomic Energy Centre in Trombay. It was because of Dr Bhabha's resolute attempts that the proposal of the Tarapur nuclear reactor was approved. The construction of the Tarapur project was looked after by Raja Ramanna at the behest of Dr Bhabha. Dr Ramanna carried out his responsibility very well. After the death of Dr Bhabha, Dr Ramanna became his worthy successor.

In 1983, he was appointed the chairman of the Atomic Energy Commission and the secretary of the Atomic Energy Department by the Government of India. On 31 January 1987, he relinquished both posts. Then with financial assistance from France, Dr Ramanna and Tata constituted the National Institute of Science, Bangalore.

Dr Ramanna was born on 28 January 1925 in Mysore, Karnataka. His father, B. Ramanna, worked at the court of Mysore. His mother, Rukmini Amma, was the daughter of the district judge. First he was called Krishnaraj, later he was called Raja. Raja Ramanna has three brothers and two sisters and is the youngest of six siblings. He died on 24 September 2004 and left a trail of technological innovations to be pursued for a global presence.

Dr A.P.J. Abdul Kalam

**Father of India's Missile Programme/
President of India**

(Born 1931)

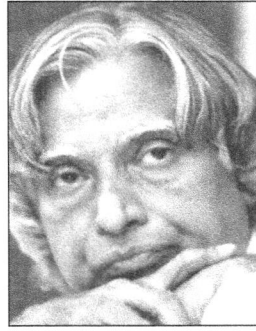

Friends and associates of Avul Pakir Jainulabdeen Abdul Kalam say that he may not be 100 per cent, but he is at least 200 per cent Indian. He has helped India build its missile muscle. He developed and successfully launched *Agni* and *Prithvi*, the two indigenously developed ballistic missiles that brought both China and Pakistan within India's missile range. But this scientist did not develop the missiles for the country's offensive purposes, but to strengthen its defence. The world now recognises India as a potent force.

Abdul Kalam was born into a Tamil Muslim family in a town named Dhanushkodi in district Rameswaram of Tamil Nadu in 1931. His father rented boats to fishermen. His quest for knowledge was inspired by one of his relatives who had a newspaper agency. Newspapers from around the country came to Rameswaram and Abdul Kalam used to gather news and information from them. This instilled in him the desire to seek knowledge. Abdul Kalam's father was a religious person and his mother was a woman with respect for traditional values. His parents and the serene atmosphere of Rameswaram left a deep impact on young Abdul Kalam's mind.

Initially Abdul Kalam studied in Rameswaram. After completing his twelfth class examinations from St Joseph's College in Tiruchirapalli, he wished to study engineering. So he joined the Madras Institute of Technology. At one time he nursed the desire of becoming a pilot. He started his career with the Defence Research and Development Organisation (DRDO) in 1958. He later moved on to the Indian Space Research Organisation (ISRO) in 1963. He helped India launch the 35-kg *Rohini I* satellite on a low-earth orbit with the help of Satellite Launch Vehicle III in July 1981. After being associated with ISRO for 19 years, he again moved to DRDO in 1982. It was Dr Raja Ramanna who asked him to take charge of India's Integrated Guided Missile Development Programme. Here he developed the short-range and intermediate-range ballistic missiles *Prithvi* and *Agni*.

Kalam led India's successful underground nuclear weapons' tests, which were held in May 1998.

He has also written four books: *Wings of Fire, India 2020 – A Vision for the New Millennium, My Journey* and *Ignited Minds – Unleashing the Power Within India.*

Abdul Kalam is a multifaceted personality. Apart from being a scientist, he is also a musician. He plays the Rudra Veena. He was honoured with the Padma Bhushan in 1981. He was honoured with the Bharat Ratna, the country's highest civilian award, in 1997. He was President of India from July 2002 to July 2007.

Dr Kalam is currently a visiting professor at Indian Institute of Management Ahmedabad, Chancellor of Indian Institute of Space Science and Technology, Thiruvananthapuram, professor of Aerospace Engineering at Anna University, Chennai, visiting professor of Indian Institute of Management, Indore and senior faculty member at many other academic and research institutions in India.

Miscellaneous

Jamnalal Bajaj

Freedom Fighter, Social Worker and Industrialist

(1889–1942)

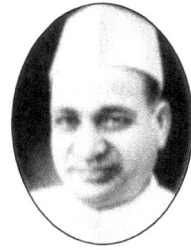

Jamnalal Bajaj was the founding father of the Bajaj Group. The adopted 'fifth' son of Mahatma Gandhi, and the 'merchant prince' who held the wealth he created in trust for the people of his country. Trust – a simple word that contains a whole philosophy handed down by Jamnalal Bajaj to his successors. He valued honesty over profit, actions over words and common good over individual gain.

Jamnalal was born on 4 November 1889, at Kasi-Ka-Bas village in Jaipur State (now the state of Rajasthan). His father Kaniram was a poor man. His mother's name was Brindibai. Jamnalal's father Kaniram had a distant but millionaire relation named Seth Bachhraj of Wardha. He had a widowed daughter-in-law who had no issue. Seth Bachhraj accompanied by his wife Sadibai once visited Kaniram's house, when they were looking for a suitable child for adoption in the family.

Attracted by Jamnalal, Sadibai asked Brindibai to allow her to adopt the child. With utmost reluctance, Jamnalal was allowed to go to Seth Bachhraj as his adopted son, at the age of four. Kaniram stoutly resisted Seth Bachhraj's offer to compensate him for this adoption and asked him to sink a well for the village in lieu of this gesture.

Jamnalal was married at the age of 13 to Jankidevi, daughter of Seth Girdharilal Jijodia of Jaora in Indore State (now the state of Madhya Pradesh). Seth Girdharilal was a wealthy businessman of Jaora. Jankidevi was then only nine years old. The marriage was a typical case of child marriage, so common in those days.

From 1896, when Jamnalal was seven, he was sent to school. He picked up the three Rs and acquired a nodding acquaintance with the English language. His education was through the medium of Marathi, but he achieved workable mastery over Gujarati, Hindi and English as he grew in years.

Jamnalal felt attracted to a number of eminent leaders in public life. He met Pandit Madan Mohan Malaviya. He spent some time with Rabindranath Tagore. He came in contact with Lokmanya Tilak whose journal, *Kesari*, he had been reading since childhood. He appreciated the assertive tone of Tilak's writings. But Jamnalal's spiritual thirst for a guide and guru could only be slaked by Gandhiji.

After the death of Seth Bachhraj, Jamnalal always felt that he had no moral right to enjoy the wealth. He kept his wealth as a 'trust'. In 1908 Jamnalal became an Honorary Magistrate. Ten years later he was given the title of Rai Bahadur. In 1915 he met Gandhiji and felt that he had at last found his spiritual guide. Gandhiji was also attracted to this earnest young man.

In 1920 Jamnalal took a momentous decision which was to change the whole course of his life. He decided to request Gandhiji to treat him as his 'fifth son'. Gandhiji was at first surprised by this strange request, but he gladly agreed to it.

He functioned as the Treasurer of the Indian National Congress practically throughout his life. In 1921 he joined the Non-cooperation Movement and founded the Satyagraha Ashram at Wardha under the guidance of Acharya Vinoba Bhave. In this very year he surrendered the title of Rai Bahadur in pursuance of a resolution passed by the Congress.

In 1923 Jamnalal Bajaj led the National Flag Satyagraha at Nagpur and was sentenced to 18 months' imprisonment. In 1924 he founded the Gandhi Seva Sangh. He also founded the Sasta Sahitya Mandal, which now has its head office in Delhi. It publishes cheap national books in Hindi.

Jamnalal Bajaj also carried on his noble work for the uplift of Harijans. He became the Secretary of the Anti-untouchability Committee of the Indian National Congress and conducted incessant propaganda in favour of the right of Harijans to enter temples. In 1928 he threw open his own Lakshminarayan Temple at Wardha to the Harijans. In 1930 he was elected leader of the Salt Satyagraha Camp at Vile Parle, Bombay.

In 1936 Jamnalal Bajaj gave Segaon village as a gift to Gandhiji who named it 'Sevagram' and founded his ashram there. In 1938 he was elected president of the Jaipur State Praja Mandal. In 1939 he was interned in Jaipur in consequence of the satyagraha campaign in the State for democratic rights. In 1941 he was arrested for anti-war propaganda during the Individual Civil Disobedience Movement. In 1941 he founded the Gouseva Sangha at Wardha for the service of cows.

On 11 February 1942 Jamnalal Bajaj died all of a sudden on account of haemorrhage due to high blood pressure. Mahatma Gandhi in his article in the *Harijan* after the death of Jamnalal Bajaj wrote: "Never was a mortal blessed with a 'son' like him… There is hardly any activity of mine in which I did not receive his full-hearted co-operation and in which it did not prove to be of the greatest value."

Amartya Kumar Sen

Renowned Economist

(Born 1933)

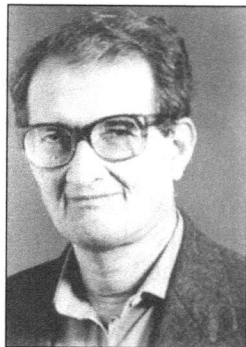

D r Amartya Kumar Sen, noted economist and philosopher, defied some of the popular 'theories' or 'laws' of economics. And when the Royal Swedish Academy awarded him the Nobel Prize in Economic Sciences for 1998, it recognised his work, especially his studies on famines and his "key contributions to welfare economics". He was the first Asian economist and the sixth Indian to receive the Nobel Prize.

According to well-known British economist Thomas Malthus famine, disease and war were the result of overpopulation. But when Amartya Sen analysed the causes of famine and starvation, he came to the conclusion that shortage of food supply was not just the cause of famine, other factors also contributed to it. Perhaps he was inspired to take up economics because he was himself a witness to the Bengal Famine of 1943. He believed that the famine was the result of man himself rather than natural causes. As a young boy of ten then, he recalled, "The streets were full of emaciated looking faces and people were dying in very large numbers. It made me think about what causes famine. Thirty years later, I was still quite haunted by the memories of that period."

Amartya Kumar Sen was born at Shantiniketan, as his father was working there. In fact he was given the name 'Amartya' or 'the one who deserves immortality' by none other than Rabindranath Tagore himself. Rabindranath Tagore had predicted that the child would go on to earn a lot of fame and recognition for himself and the country.

He studied at Shantiniketan and topped in his intermediate examination. In 1953, he joined Presidency College in Calcutta for his graduation in economics. Then he went to England and joined Cambridge University for his post-graduation and doctorate. When he came back to India, he joined Jadavpur University as professor of economics. He was then just 24.

In 1963 he moved on to Delhi School of Economics (DSE), where he taught for eight years. His fellow professors were V.K.R.V. Rao and K.N. Raj, who were renowned economists. He was associated with DSE till 1971. Then he shifted base to England and joined London School of Economics. He later moved on to Oxford as professor of economics and philosophy. He stayed there for almost a decade before taking over as Master of Trinity College at Cambridge.

Dr Sen has authored about 21 books and over 200 research papers and articles. He has tried to analyse the relation between poverty and famine. Basing his research on the Bengal Famine of 1943, he came to the conclusion that famines are actually man-made catastrophes and not natural disasters. According to him, the famine was the result of the poverty prevalent in the area. The poor did not have the buying capacity. When the prices of food grains soared and the poor did not get a raise in their salaries or supplement their income in some other way, they had to starve. Dr Sen also proved that the main reason behind poverty was illiteracy.

Amartya Sen was married to Navnita Dev in 1960. She is a famous Bengali writer. They were divorced in 1974. They have two children. In 1977, he married a student of DSE named Eva, but she died in 1985. Then he went to England to join London School of Economics. When he joined Trinity College, he met Emma Rothschild who was also teaching there. He later married her.

In recognition of his work, in January 1999, the Indian Government honoured him with India's highest civilian award, the Bharat Ratna.

Tenzing Norgay

Pioneer Conqueror of Everest

(1914–1986)

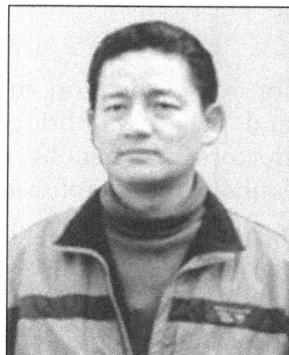

Standing 8,848m tall, Mt Everest in the Himalayan mountain ranges is the highest mountain peak in the world. On 29 May 1953, Tenzing Norgay, along with New Zealand's Edmund Hillary, became the first to conquer Everest. For more than 50 years, expeditions were being undertaken to conquer the world's highest peak. Many even gave up their lives vying for the honour of being the first to conquer Everest. It remained insurmountable till 1953, when Norgay hoisted the tricolour on the peak.

Tenzing Norgay – originally Namgyal Wangdi, meaning, 'Wealthy, Fortunate Follower of Religion' – was born on 15 May 1914 at Solo Khumbu in Nepal. No one could have guessed that the eleventh child amongst 13 children of an unknown man who lived at Thami village in the district south of Everest could go on to create history. The village was inhabited by *sherpas* (Nepalese people skilled in mountain climbing who primarily work as porters for mountaineers).

As a young boy he ran away from home and settled in Darjeeling, West Bengal. In 1935, he joined Sir Eric Shipton's expedition to Everest as a porter. After the Second World War, he became a *sirdar*, or organiser of porters.

In 1953, he accompanied the British Everest expedition as a *sirdar*. He formed the second summit pair with Edmund Hillary. On 29 May 1953, at 11:30 a.m. they reached the summit. Tenzing Norgay spent 15 minutes on the summit. As a devout Buddhist, he left an offering of food on the summit.

He was considered a hero both in India and Nepal. A controversy brewed about his nationality, but Tenzing silenced it by saying:

"It's true that I was born in Nepal, but was reared and looked after by India."

Pt Nehru congratulated him and helped him set the Mountaineering Training Institute and appointed him the director. He served the Institute till the end. He shared his experiences with aspiring mountaineers at the Institute. When the Institute was inaugurated, Pt Nehru remarked, "This Institute will now produce thousands of Tenzings."

Tenzing believed that for achieving success in any arduous job, one should display immense courage, perseverance, intellect and the potential to face difficult situations. It is because of these inborn qualities in him that Tenzing went on to conquer Everest.

Tenzing was awarded the Padma Bhushan by the President. The Queen of England bestowed on him the George Medal while the Nepal Government conferred on him the title *Nepal Tara* (Star of Nepal).

Tenzing Norgay died on 9 May 1986 in Darjeeling.

Sam Manekshaw

India's First Field Marshal

(1914–2008)

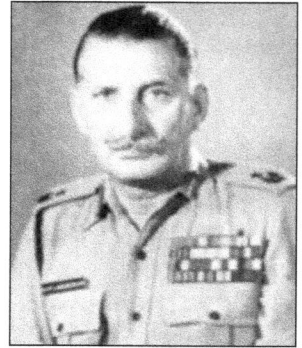

G eneral Manekshaw's name figures prominently in the list of important personalities of the 20th Century. This is because during his tenure in the army, many critical moments came up where the Indian Army had the chance to display their undaunted courage, valour and loyalty. The Indian Army is considered one of the outstanding armies of the world.

Sam Hormuzji Framji Jamshedji Manekshaw, popularly known as Sam Manekshaw, was born in Amritsar on 13 April 1914. Serving in the army had been a passion that he nurtured from childhood. After passing out from Sherwood College, a school in Nainital, he appeared for the army entrance examination. He was one among the 15 candidates finally selected from 12,000 applicants. In 1934, at the age of 20, he passed out from the Indian Military Academy at Dehradun.

On his first assignment, he had to fight the Pathans in the North-West Frontier Province. When the Second World War was at its peak, Sam Manekshaw was sent to Rangoon (now Yangon) to defend Burma (now Myanmar) against the Japanese. The Indian and Japanese army had a confrontation at Sitang Bridge. If the Japanese had been successful in capturing the bridge, it would have become easier to enter India. So Indian forces had to defend it with all their might. Young Manekshaw showed undaunted courage and thwarted the efforts of the Japanese. In the event, the young Captain received six bullets in his stomach. It could have been the end of his dream, but he made an amazing recovery and was awarded the Military Cross for his gallantry.

In 1947, when India was attacked by Pakistani mercenaries, Sam Manekshaw was given the onus of stopping them from advancing on Indian soil. Manekshaw was a good strategist and always drew his plan of action and discussed it with the concerned minister. However, when he discussed the Chinese incursion into India in 1959, his strategy was rejected by the then defence minister V.K. Krishna Menon. But during the Chinese aggression, Sam Manekshaw was asked to thwart it.

Even in the 1971 war with Pakistan, Sam Manekshaw displayed immense valour and led India to a tremendous victory.

For his commendable services to the nation, he was awarded Padma Vibhushan in 1972 and also made the first Indian Field Marshal on 1 January 1973. Throughout his scintillating career that spanned over 40 years, he overawed generals, statesmen, politicians and soldiers alike. The British Commander-in-Chief of the Indian Army during the Second World War, General Sir Roy Butcher, while praising Manekshaw's dedication and valour, said, "The very best staff officer I ever had."

After retirement, Manekshaw had settled down at Coonoor in the Nilgiris. He keeps himself busy by tending cows, bees, poultry and tea plantations. Be it on the battlefront or homefront, for a strict disciplinarian, life knows no difference.

Sam Manekshaw died at the Military Hospital in Wellington (Tamil Nadu) on 27 June 2008 at the age of 94 due to complications arising out of pneumonia. Adjacent to his wife's grave, he was laid to rest in Ootacamund, Tamil Nadu, with full military honours,

Salim Ali

The Birdman of India

(1896–1987)

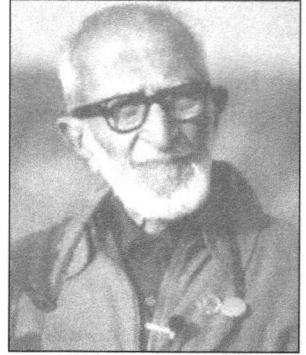

Dr Salim Ali was one of the world's leading ornithologists. Ali's passion for bird-watching was so strong that he would travel to even the remotest places to pursue his hobby, earning him the title of the Birdman of India.

Dr Salim Ali was born on 12 November 1896 in Bombay. He was initiated into this hobby because of an incident that happened when he was just ten. He shot a sparrow with his air-gun, but the bird seemed unusual. It had a yellow patch on the throat. He wanted to identify it, so he went to the Bombay Natural History Society for this. He was surprised that there were about a dozen species of sparrows and this particular species was one.

Salim Ali wanted to take up ornithology – the study of birds and bird behaviour – so he went to Berlin to study it. Back in India he observed birds in their natural habitat. He made many new and interesting observations about birds. In *The Book of Indian Birds*, he wrote about his observations and gave a boost to bird-watching in India. He co-authored *The Handbook of the Birds of India and Pakistan* with Dr S. Dillon Ripley, which documents observations about more than 2,000 birds in the subcontinent.

In 1976 he was honoured with the Padma Vibhushan. This year, he also won the J. Paul Getty Wildlife Conservation Prize. Dr Salim Ali encouraged bird-watching among the people. He said, "All that you need is an inexpensive pair of binoculars, a notebook, a pencil and an ample stock of patience and dedication." He was an active campaigner for bird conservation in the country.

The renowned ornithologist passed away on 27 July 1987.

Dr Verghese Kurien

Father of the White Revolution

(Born 1921)

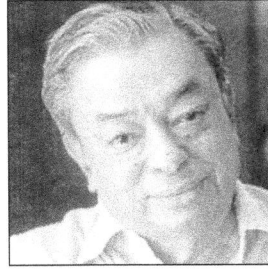

Dr Verghese Kurien is the man behind the success of Operation Flood, the movement that helped treble the country's milk production, making it self-sufficient in the production of milk and milk products.

India is a land of villages and a majority of the farmers of these villages keep milch cows and buffaloes. They sell the milk in towns and cities. India leads in the production of milk, but as the villagers were not working in cooperation with each other, they did not benefit from the sale of the milk. This also affected the production of milk. Verghese Kurien formed a co-operative society of such farmers that not only took care of poor, marginal farmers, but also inspired them to expand their business. In this way he laid the foundation of the dairy industry.

Kurien studied engineering at the Michigan University in America. Back in India in 1949, he took up a job at Anand in Gujarat. His dream of improving the farmers' lives was fulfilled by the milk co-operatives. Today, the Anand Co-operative is a well-known industry and the name AMUL is famous the world over.

Very few people know who really was the inspiration behind the co-operative movement. It was Sardar Patel who first worked towards the betterment of the farmers of the area. Later he entrusted the work of improving the living standards of villagers of Kaira and the adjoining areas to Tribhuvandas Patel, who mobilised milk producers into cooperatives.

When Verghese Kurien went to Anand, he changed the concept of dairying. He established a network of veterinary services and cattle-breeding centres. In 1965 he took over as the head of the National Dairy Development Board. He proposed establishing the 'Anand Pattern' all over the country. In 1970 came Operation Flood – a movement that involved 170 million people. It has the credit of being the largest dairy development network in the world. Around six million dairy owners belonging to 75,000 village cooperatives supply milk to 500 towns and cities. Operation Flood has helped stabilise milk prices in the country and ensure the supply of fresh, hygienic milk. India has ceased to depend on milk imports and the co-operative provides a source of regular income to the farmers. Apart from whole and skimmed milk, Anand produces condensed milk, butter, cheese and cheese spreads.

Verghese Kurien has been honoured with several national and international awards. The awards include the Padma Shri, the Padma Bhushan, the Magsaysay Award, the World Food Prize and the Padma Vibhushan. But Verghese Kurien is a modest man. He says that he owes his success to the farmers of Gujarat.

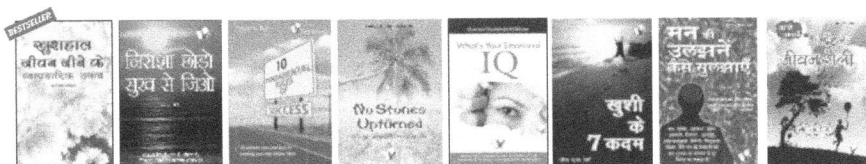

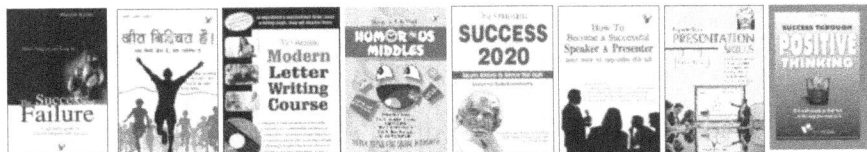

Also Available
in Hindi

Also Available
in Hindi

Also Available
in Kannada, Tamil

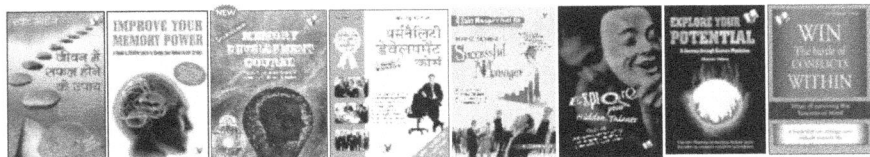

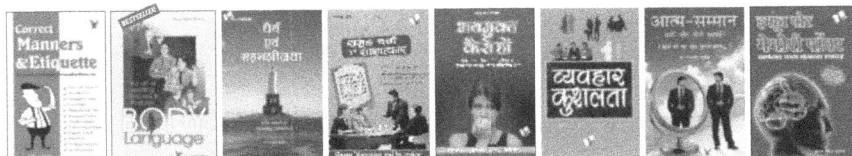

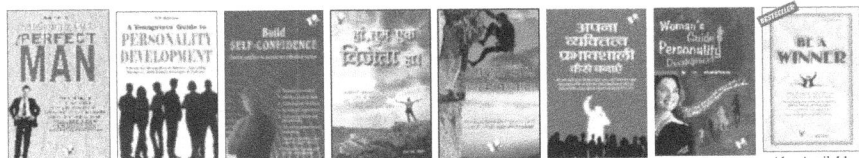

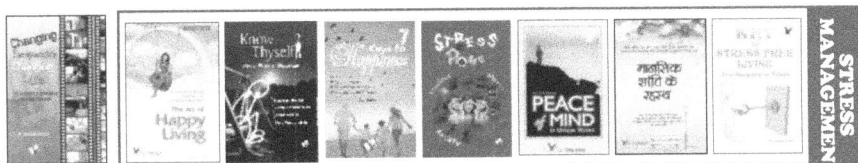

Also Available
in Kannada

Also Available
in Kannada

STRESS MANAGEMENT

All books available at www.vspublishers.com

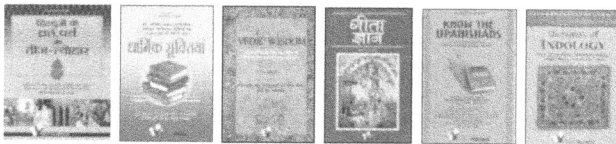

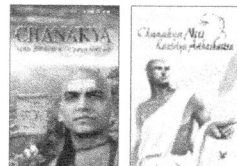

Also Available
in Hindi, Kannada

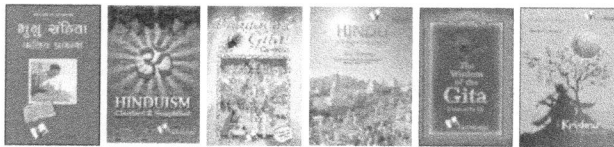

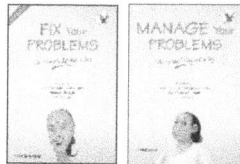

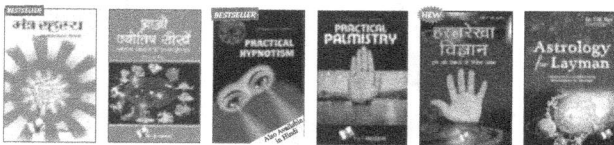

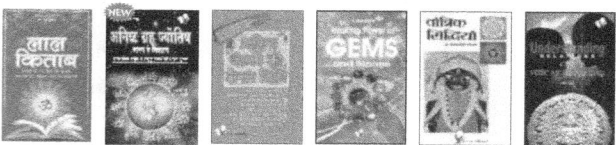

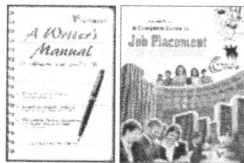

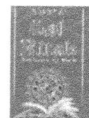

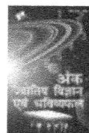

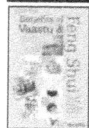

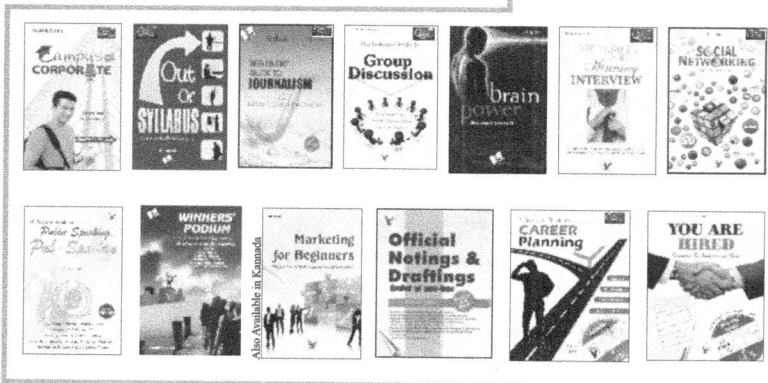

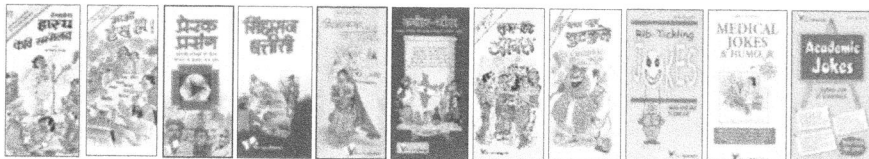

Also Available
in Hindi, Kannada

Also Available in Kannada

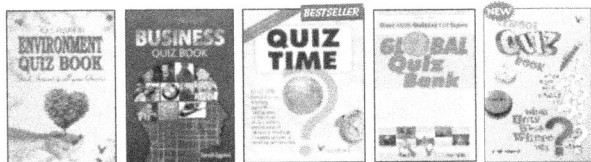
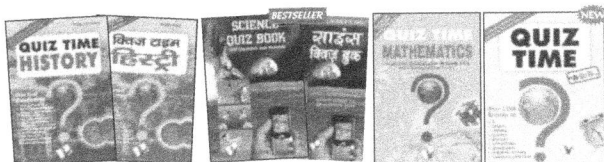
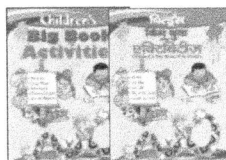
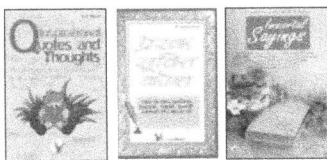
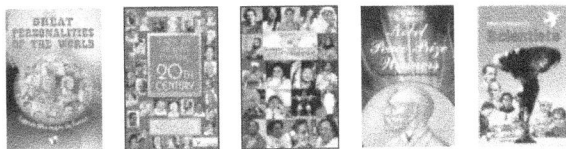
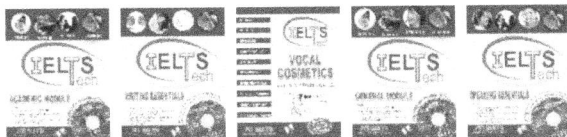
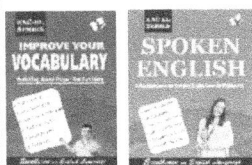
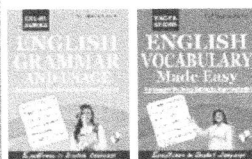
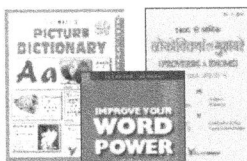
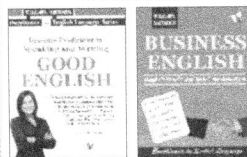
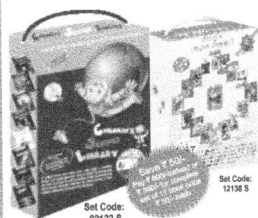
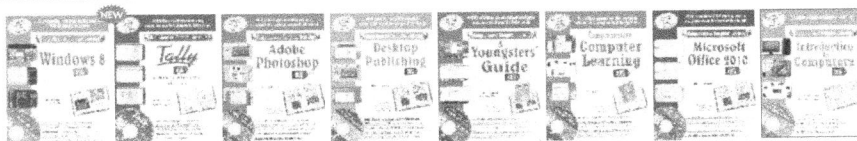

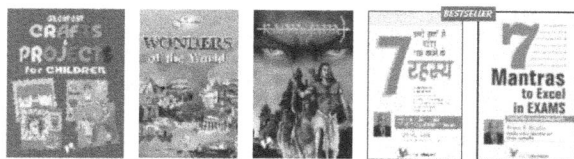
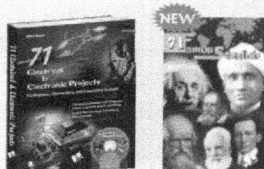
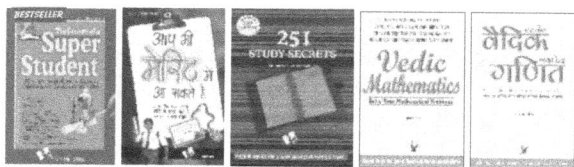
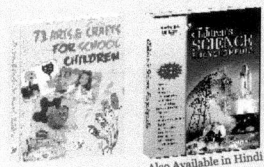
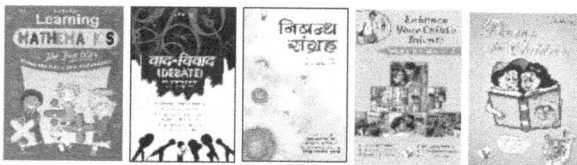
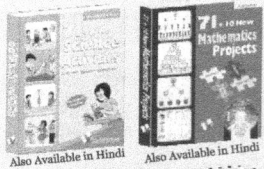
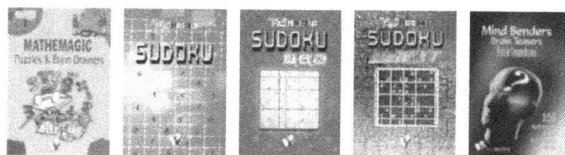
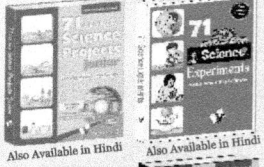
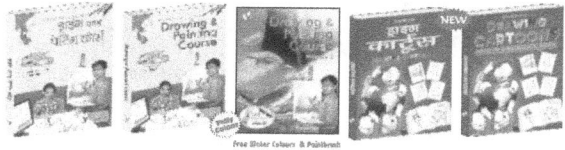
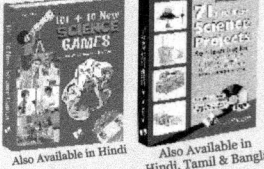
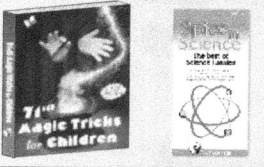
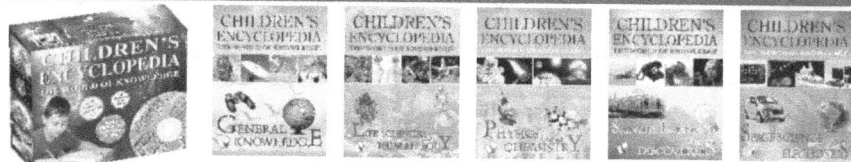